JESSICA TELLEZ

Quick Fit: "Efficient Workouts for Busy Lives"

First edition

This book was professionally typeset on Reedsy.
Find out more at reedsy.com

Contents

1

Introduction

Quick Fit: "Efficient Workouts for Busy Lives"

Facing the constant juggle of a demanding career and personal life, I realized the necessity for efficient, effective workouts that fit into busy schedules. This led to the birth of Quick Fit – a guide to swift, impactful exercise routines tailored for busy adults. This book offers practical, time-saving strategies to maintain fitness amidst a hectic lifestyle, addressing the common challenge of finding time for exercise and debunking the myth that workouts must be extended to be effective. At the core of Quick Fit are concise workouts designed to be completed in 30 minutes or less, utilizing high-intensity interval training (HIIT), bodyweight exercises, and efficient strength training to yield maximum results swiftly. These routines offer several benefits: they are time-efficient, adaptable to any setting, suitable for all fitness levels, and effective in enhancing strength, cardiovascular health, and mood. Structured in an easy-to-navigate format, the book introduces quick workouts and their scientific backing, followed by diverse routines with detailed instructions and illustrations, covering different muscle groups and full-body exercises. A stretching and recovery section ensures a balanced fitness approach, promoting injury prevention and flexibility. Drawing from extensive personal training experience and a passion for fitness, I've crafted these time-efficient exercise solutions to help busy individuals balance time constraints with fitness goals. While not a cure-all, quick workouts are a potent tool for steadily improving strength, endurance, and overall health when consistently incorporated into one's routine. Embrace the Quick Fit approach: integrate these flexible, enjoyable, and effective workouts into your life, regardless of your schedule. Experiment with various routines to find what suits you best, and relish the journey to a fitter, healthier you. Let's dive in!

2

Chapter 1: Getting Started with Quick Workouts

Years ago, I was overwhelmed by the challenge of incorporating lengthy workouts into my busy schedule. However, after experimenting with quick workouts on a friend's advice, I noticed a significant improvement in my energy levels, strength, and stress reduction. This journey ignited my interest in the science behind quick workouts, which I've explored in this book. # 1.1 The Benefits of Quick Workouts High-Intensity Interval Training (HIIT) epitomizes the efficiency of quick workouts. By alternating between intense activity bursts and brief rest periods, HIIT proves to be as effective, if not more, than prolonged cardio sessions. Studies from the National Center for Biotechnology Information (NCBI) highlight HIIT's ability to enhance metabolic health and exercise capacity with minimal time investment. Such efficiency extends to various short, intense exercises, offering similar benefits. Quick workouts not only save time but also provide substantial health benefits. They improve cardiovascular health, muscle tone, strength, flexibility, and mobility while boosting mental well-being through endorphin release.

Contrary to common myths, research reveals that short workouts are effective for all fitness levels and can be done anywhere with minimal or no equipment. Consistency with this type of workout yields long-term health benefits, as the cumulative effects of small, daily exercises accumulate over time. For successful integration, consider scheduling exercises during breaks or early mornings. This habit ensures steady progress without overwhelming your schedule. # 1.2 Understanding Your Fitness Level Before Starting: Assess your fitness level to tailor workouts effectively, minimizing injury risks and burnout. Self-assessment quizzes and basic fitness tests, like push-ups or sit-and-reach tests, can gauge your physical condition. Whether you're a beginner, intermediate, or advanced exerciser, understanding your starting point helps you set realistic goals and choose appropriate workouts. Gradually ramping up the difficulty of your workouts guarantees ongoing progress and keeps you motivated. # 1.3 Essential Gear for Quick Workouts: The right equipment can elevate your workout. Key items include:

- Comfortable, moisture-wicking clothing.
- Supportive athletic shoes.
- Versatile resistance bands for both strength and flexibility training.

Additional items like yoga mats, dumbbells, or kettle bells can further diversify your routines. Cost-effective options and proper gear maintenance ensure a successful workout experience. # 1.4 Setting realistic fitness goals with the SMART criteria—Specific, Measurable, Achievable, Relevant, and Time-bound is crucial. These goals support motivation and focus, making tracking progress and remaining committed easier. Examples include aiming to improve plank hold time or increasing workout frequency. Tracking progress, adjusting goals as needed, and celebrating achievements are critical components of a successful fitness journey. Employing the SMART criteria transforms vague aspirations into clear, actionable objectives, promoting continuous progress and making fitness an attainable part of your life.

3

Chapter 2: Warm-Up and Cool down Essentials

One evening, after a long day at work, I decided to skip my usual warm-up and dive straight into my workout. Within minutes, I felt a sharp pain in my calf, forcing me to stop. That incident was a harsh reminder of the importance of warming up before any exercise. A proper warm-up is not just a formality; it's a crucial step that prepares your body for the physical demands ahead, reducing the risk of injury and enhancing your overall performance.

Quick Warm-Up Routines for Busy Schedules

Warming up is essential for several reasons. First and foremost, it increases blood flow to your muscles, ensuring they are well-oxygenated and ready for action. This heightened circulation raises the temperature of your muscles, making them more elastic and less prone to strains or tears. An excellent warm-up prepares your cardiovascular system for increased heart rate and physical exertion. It gradually elevates your heart rate, minimizing the stress on your heart and preventing sudden spikes that can be harmful, especially if you jump straight into high-intensity exercise from a passive state.

An effective warm-up should be quick yet comprehensive, incorporating light cardio, dynamic stretches, and joint mobility exercises. Begin with a minute of jumping jacks to elevate your heart rate. Then, move on to a minute of arm circles to warm your shoulders and arms. Continue with high knees for a minute to engage your core and activate your legs. Follow this with hip circles for a minute to loosen the hip joints. Conclude with a minute of dynamic lunges and alternating legs to prepare your body for the workout ahead. This streamlined 5-minute routine ensures you hit all the necessary components to increase muscle elasticity, boost circulation, and enhance joint mobility, setting a solid foundation for any exercise regimen.

Adjusting the intensity and duration of your warm-up based on your fitness level is essential to ensure it is effective and safe. You might start with lower intensity and fewer repetitions if you're a beginner. For example, you could march in place instead of high knees, lifting your knees to a comfortable height. Intermediate exercisers can maintain a moderate intensity with more repetitions, ensuring that the warm-up is challenging enough to prepare the body for a more intense workout. Advanced individuals can add movements to increase the intensity. For instance, advanced exercisers might include butt kicks or plyometric moves like jump squats in their warm-up to ensure their bodies are fully prepared for high-intensity activities.

Quiz: Assess Your Warm-Up Knowledge

1. What is the primary purpose of a warm-up?

- A) To increase muscle elasticity
- B) To prepare the cardiovascular system
- C) Both A and B

1. Which of the following is a dynamic stretch?

- A) Touching your toes and holding
- B) Arm circles
- C) Sitting and stretching your hamstrings

1. How long should a standard warm-up routine last?

- A) 2-3 minutes
- B) 5-10 minutes
- C) 15-20 minutes

Incorporating these warm-up routines into your exercise regime can significantly enhance your performance and reduce the risk of injury. Whether you're a beginner or an advanced athlete, adjusting the intensity to match your fitness level ensures that your warm-up is effective and enjoyable. This way, you can transition smoothly into your main workout, knowing that your body is well-prepared and ready to tackle the challenges ahead.

2.2 Effective Cool down Techniques

2.2 Effective Cool down Techniques: Cooling down after a workout is essential for a smooth transition back to rest, helping to minimize injury risks and facilitate recovery. It allows for a gradual decrease in heart rate, preventing the sudden drop that can stress the cardiovascular system. Cooling down also counters blood pooling in the extremities, which can lead to dizziness or fainting, by maintaining circulation and stabilizing blood pressure. Moreover, it eases muscle stiffness by allowing muscle fibers, which experience tiny tears during exercise, to return to their average length, thereby reducing post-exercise soreness. An effective cool down routine should start with light aerobic activities like walking to sustain blood flow and gradually lower the heart rate. This should be followed by static stretching, with each stretch lasting 15 to 30 seconds, which helps with muscle relaxation and restoring length.

Ending with deep breathing exercises improves muscle oxygenation, encourages relaxation, and reduces stress, helping the body and mind transition from exertion to calm. A practical 5-minute cool down might involve one minute of slow walking, followed by one minute each of a standing quad stretch and a seated forward bend to stretch the thighs, hamstrings, and lower back. Proceed with one minute of shoulder stretches to alleviate tension in the shoulders and upper back, and finish with one minute of deep breathing to relax the body entirely. Tailoring the cool down routine to individual needs is essential. Seniors may benefit from longer, gentler stretches to accommodate slower muscle relaxation. At the same time, athletes could require sport-specific stretches to focus on the most used muscles. Those with injuries should opt for low-impact movements to avoid further strain while promoting recovery. These cool down techniques ensure proper recovery post-workout, preparing the body for future exercise and maintaining a healthy, effective fitness routine. Cooling down is not merely an afterthought but a critical component of your exercise regimen.

2.3 Dynamic Stretching for Flexibility

Dynamic stretching is a vital component of any effective warm-up routine, and it differs significantly from static stretching. Static stretching involves holding a stretch for a set duration. In contrast, dynamic stretching entails moving your body parts and progressively increasing your reach, speed, or both. This type of stretching prepares your muscles for active use by mimicking the movements you'll perform during your workout. As you engage in these controlled movements, you enhance your range of motion, making your muscles more pliable and ready for exercise demands. Unlike static stretches, which are better suited for cool downs, dynamic stretches are designed to warm the body.

Incorporating dynamic stretching into your warm-up routine offers several advantages. One of the primary benefits is improved flexibility and mobility. By moving through the full range of motion, you loosen up your muscles and joints, which helps reduce muscle stiffness. This is especially important before activities that require explosive movements, such as running or jumping. Dynamic stretching enhances overall performance by increasing muscle temperature and promoting better blood flow. This prepares your body to handle the intensity of your workout, reducing the risk of injury and making your movements more efficient and effective.

Several dynamic stretches are particularly effective for warming up. Leg swings are an excellent choice. Stand on one leg and swing the other leg forward and backward, gradually increasing the height of your swing. This targets your hip flexors and hamstrings, preparing them for more intense activity. Arm circles are another great option. Extend your arms to the sides and make small circles, gradually increasing the size of the circles. This helps warm up your shoulders and upper back. Hip rotations are also beneficial. Stand with your feet shoulder-width apart and rotate your hips in a circular motion, clockwise and counterclockwise. This loosens up your hip joints and lower back. Walking lunges with a twist adds an extra layer of complexity. Step forward into a lunge, twist your torso towards your front leg, and return to the starting position. This dynamic stretch engages your legs, core, and upper body, making it a comprehensive warm-up exercise.

Incorporating dynamic stretching into your quick workouts is straightforward and highly effective. Start by performing each dynamic stretch for about 30 seconds. This ensures that your muscles have enough time to warm up without causing fatigue. Combine these stretches with light cardio activities, such as jogging in place or jumping jacks, to create a whole warm-up routine that prepares your entire body. Adjust the intensity of the stretches based on your fitness level. For beginners, start with smaller movements and gradually increase the range and speed as you become more comfortable. Intermediate exercisers can aim for moderate intensity, ensuring that each stretch is challenging but manageable. Advanced individuals can push the intensity further by incorporating more complex movements and faster speeds. The key is to listen to your body and adjust accordingly to ensure a safe and effective warm-up.

Dynamic stretching is an integral part of preparing your body for exercise. By moving through controlled, full-range movements, you enhance your flexibility, reduce muscle stiffness, and get your body ready for the demands of your workout. Whether you are a beginner or an advanced athlete, incorporating dynamic stretches into your warm-up routine can significantly improve your performance and reduce the risk of injury.

2.4 The Role of Breathing in Warm-Up and Cool down

Proper breathing techniques are crucial yet often overlooked aspects of effective warm-up and cool down routines. Correct breathing enhances oxygen flow to muscles, is vital for peak performance, and reduces the risk of muscle cramps and fatigue. During warm-ups, efficient breathing increases oxygen supply, boosts energy levels, and fosters a calm, focused mindset crucial for precise and controlled movement execution. Diaphragmatic or belly breathing into your warm-up activates total lung capacity, optimizing oxygen intake. Rhythmic breathing, which synchronizes breath with movement, such as inhaling and exhaling with squat motions, regulates breathing and is especially beneficial during intense exercise. Shifting to the cool down phase, the focus is on relaxation and recovery. Deep, slow breaths lower the heart rate and blood pressure, calming the nervous system and easing the body from exertion to relaxation. Techniques like the 4-7-8 breathing pattern, inhaling through the nose for four counts, holding for seven, and exhaling through the mouth for eight, significantly reduce stress and cultivate calmness. Alternate nostril breathing also balances the body's energy and soothes the mind. Integrating mindfulness with breathing practices elevates warm-up and cool down routines to holistic experiences. Focusing on the sensation of air flowing in and out and how it affects both physical and mental states centers the mind and increases workout engagement. Mindful breathing and gentle movements such as slow stretches or yoga poses create a comprehensive cool down routine that promotes physical and mental recovery, enriching the overall fitness experience and deepening the body-mind connection. By emphasizing proper breathing throughout warm-up and cool down, the effectiveness of these routines is significantly improved. Proper techniques ensure adequate oxygen delivery to muscles, reducing injury risk and improving performance. At the same time, mindful breathing enhances relaxation and mental clarity, making workouts more enjoyable and productive. Incorporating these techniques, regardless of fitness level, leads to a balanced and holistic exercise experience.

4

Chapter 3: Core Strength in Minutes

I remember being excited when I was invited to a beach vacation with my family; that excitement quickly turned into anxiety as I thought about wearing a swimsuit. Despite my busy schedule, I was determined to strengthen my core and improve my confidence. That's when I discovered the power of quick core workouts. In just minutes a day, I started to see results. This chapter focuses on helping you achieve similar results with a minimal time investment.

5-Minute Core Blast

A quick core workout can yield significant results if done correctly. The core is the powerhouse of your body. It supports nearly every movement, from bending to lifting to sitting straight. A strong core stabilizes your body, improves balance, and prevents injuries. When you think about core exercises, long sessions at the gym might come to mind. However, you can build a strong core with just a few intense minutes each day. This 5-minute routine is designed to efficiently target all significant core muscles, making it perfect for busy lives.

Let's jump into the routine. Start with one minute of bicycle crunches. Lie on your back, place your hands behind your head, and bring your knees towards your chest. Alternate touching your elbow to the opposite knee in a pedaling motion. This exercise engages your rectus abdominis and obliques, working both the front and sides of your core. Next, proceed with one minute of Russian twists. Sit on the floor with your knees bent and lean back slightly while keeping your back straight. Hold your hands together before you and twist your torso from side to side, touching the floor beside you with each twist. This movement targets the obliques and improves rotational strength.

The third exercise is one minute of leg raises. Lie flat on your back with your legs extended. Lift your legs towards the ceiling, keeping them straight, then lower them back down without touching the floor. This exercise focuses on the lower abs and hip flexors. Follow this with one minute of mountain climbers. Start in a plank position and quickly alternate, bringing your knees towards your chest as if running in place. This dynamic movement engages your core and increases your heart rate, adding cardio to the workout. Finally, end with one minute of a plank hold. Assume a forearm plank position, maintaining a straight line from head to heels. This static hold works the entire core, including the deep stabilizing muscles.

The advantages of this 5-minute core routine are numerous. First and foremost, it improves core stability. A stable core supports your spine and pelvis, enhancing overall body control and reducing the risk of injuries. Enhanced muscle tone is another benefit. Regularly working your core muscles will lead to a more defined midsection. Better posture is a natural result of a strong core. When your core muscles are engaged and strong, they support your spine, helping you stand and sit taller. Additionally, this routine can increase your metabolic rate. Engaging large muscle groups, like those in the core, boosts your metabolism, helping you burn more calories even at rest.

Consistency is vital to seeing these benefits. Make sure to perform this routine regularly to achieve the best results. Aim to integrate it into your daily or weekly workout schedule. You might start doing it every other day, gradually increasing the frequency as your strength and endurance improve. Maintaining motivation can sometimes be challenging, especially with a busy schedule. To keep yourself engaged, consider setting specific goals, such as increasing the number of repetitions or holding the plank for longer. Tracking your progress in a fitness journal can also be highly motivating. Seeing your improvements on paper provides a sense of accomplishment and encourages you to keep going.

This 5-minute core blast is a powerful tool in your fitness arsenal. It's quick, efficient, and practical, ideal for busy adults. Incorporating this routine into your schedule will build a stronger core, improve your posture, and boost your overall fitness. Consistency and dedication will bring you closer to your fitness goals, one minute at a time.

Plank Variations for a Strong Core

The plank exercise is a staple in core training for good reason. It engages multiple muscle groups simultaneously, making it an efficient way to build strength and stability. You activate your abs, glutes, shoulders, and legs by holding your body straight from head to heels. This full-body engagement improves balance and overall strength. The plank is a versatile exercise that can be adjusted to fit any fitness level, making it accessible for beginners and challenging for advanced athletes.

For beginners, the forearm plank is a great starting point. Begin by positioning your forearms on the ground, elbows aligned directly under your shoulders. Extend your legs behind you, resting on the balls of your feet. Keep your body straight, engaging your core to prevent your hips from sagging. This variation reduces the strain on your wrists and still provides a solid core workout. As you progress, you can transition to more challenging variations, such as the side plank. This intermediate exercise targets the obliques and improves lateral stability. Start by lying on your side, then lift your body off the ground, supporting yourself on one forearm and the side of one foot. Hold for a set duration before switching sides.

Advanced practitioners might enjoy the plank with a leg lift. Begin in a standard plank position, then lift one leg off the ground, keeping it straight. Hold for a few seconds, then switch legs. This variation increases the intensity, engaging even more muscle groups and challenging your balance. Plank jacks are an excellent choice for those looking for a high-intensity option. Start in a plank position and jump your feet out to the sides, then back together, similar to a jumping jack. This dynamic movement works your core and boosts cardio, making it a great addition to any workout.

Maintaining proper form and technique is crucial to prevent injuries and maximize the benefits of your plank exercises. Always keep your body in a straight line from head to heels. Engage your core throughout the exercise to avoid sagging or arching your back, which can strain your lower spine. Focus on keeping your shoulders aligned with your elbows and your neck in a neutral position. If you feel your form slipping, taking a short break and resetting is better than continuing with poor alignment. Proper form ensures you effectively target the intended muscle groups and avoid unnecessary strain.

To keep your plank routine engaging and motivating, consider incorporating plank challenges. A 30-day plank challenge is an excellent way to increase your endurance gradually. Start with holding a plank for 10 seconds on the first day, then add 5-10 seconds each day until you reach several minutes by the end of the month. This progressive approach helps build strength and stamina without overwhelming you. Another fun option is a weekly plank variations challenge. Each day of the week, try a different plank variation, such as the forearm plank, side plank, or plank jacks. This variety keeps your workouts exciting and targets different muscle groups.

Partner plank challenges can add a social element to your workouts, making them more enjoyable. Pair up with a friend or family member and take turns holding planks while the other person times you. You can also try synchronized plank exercises, such as doing plank jacks together or passing a small object back and forth while holding a plank. These partner activities make the workout more fun and provide an extra layer of motivation and accountability.

Incorporating these plank variations into your routine will help you build a robust and stable core. Whether you're a beginner or an advanced athlete, there's a plank exercise that suits your needs. You'll keep your workouts engaging and effective by maintaining proper form and challenging yourself with different variations and challenges.

3.3 Abdominal Workouts Without Equipment

Quick and Effective Abdominal Workouts:

Abdominal exercises are uniquely practical and don't require equipment, allowing you to work out anywhere from home to vacation spots without needing gym memberships or expensive gear.

Here are some practical exercises that only require your body weight:

- Crunches target the upper abdominal muscles. Lie on your back with your knees bent and feet flat. Hands should be behind your head, elbows wide. Engage your core, lifting your shoulder blades off the ground without pulling on your neck.
- Reverse crunches; shift the focus to the lower abs. In the same starting position, lift your hips, drawing your knees towards your chest.
- Flutter kicks work both abs and hip flexors. Lying on your back, legs straight and slightly lifted, kick your legs alternately.
- V-ups are more intense, targeting upper and lower abs together. Start flat, lifting arms and legs to form a "V."
- Hollow holds; build endurance. Lie back, extend arms and legs, and lift, forming a hollow shape, pressing your lower back into the floor. The technique is vital: engage your core, avoid momentum, and focus on controlled movements. For example, lift and lower slowly during crunches to maximize muscle engagement.

A No-Equipment Abdominal Routine:

- Crunches: 3 sets of 15, warming up the upper abs.
- Reverse Crunches: 3 sets of 12, targeting lower abs.
- Flutter Kicks: 3 sets of 20 kicks, engaging the core.
- V-ups: 3 sets of 10 for a comprehensive abdominal challenge.
- Hollow Holds: 3 sets of 20-second holds, building endurance. Rest 30-60 seconds between sets.

Core Exercises for Beginners for those new or returning to fitness, starting with low-impact, simple exercises are important to build core strength without strain. Here are some examples:

- Dead bugs: engage the core with minimal stress. You are lying down, extending your arms, and bending your knees. Alternately lower the opposite arm and leg, keeping your back pressed down.
- Bird dogs improve balance and core strength. Extend the opposite arm and leg on all fours, keeping your back flat.
- Seated knee tucks; target lower abs; sitting with legs extended, lean back, lift legs, and tuck knees to chest.
- Standing side bends are ideal for the obliques; stand and slowly bend side to side, engaging your core. Progress by increasing repetitions, adding holds or pulses, or incorporating more challenging variations to enhance muscle engagement.

Beginner Routine:

- Dead Bugs: 2 sets of 10 for core stability. -
- Bird Dogs: 2 sets of 10, improving balance. -
- Seated Knee Tucks: 2 sets of 15, focusing on lower abs.

- Standing Side Bends: 2 sets of 20 engaging obliques. Listen to your body, adjusting intensity as needed. Starting with these exercises lays a foundation for strength and stability, paving the way for more advanced workouts. A strong core supports overall fitness and daily activities.

5

Chapter 4: Lower Body Power

I remember struggling to keep up with my kids during a simple game of tag. My legs felt weak, and I realized that neglecting lower body strength impacted my daily life. That experience was a wake-up call, prompting me to focus on building more muscular legs. I quickly discovered the profound impact leg strength has on overall fitness and daily activities. Strong legs are the foundation of a stable and active body.

Leg strength is crucial for several reasons. First, it supports body stability. Your legs bear the weight of your entire body and provide the foundation for balance and coordination. Whether standing, walking, or lifting something heavy, strong legs help you maintain a stable and controlled posture. This stability reduces the risk of falls and injuries, especially as you age.

Additionally, strong legs enhance athletic performance. Many sports and physical activities rely heavily on leg strength, from running and jumping to cycling and swimming. Powerful legs can improve your speed, agility, and endurance, giving you a competitive edge. Moreover, leg strength is associated with a reduced risk of injury. Engaging in regular leg-strengthening exercises helps protect your joints and ligaments, reducing the likelihood of strains and sprains. Finally, strong legs improve functional mobility. Everyday tasks such as climbing stairs, carrying groceries, or playing with your children become more accessible and more enjoyable when your legs are strong and resilient.

Incorporating leg exercises into your routine can be something other than fancy equipment or a gym membership. You can do several quick and practical leg exercises at home with just your body weight. Body weight squats are a fantastic exercise that targets your quads, hamstrings, and glutes. To perform a body weight squat:

1. Stand with your feet shoulder-width apart.
2. Lower your body as if sitting back into a chair, keeping your chest and knees aligned with your toes.
3. Push through your heels to return to the starting position.

Lunges are another excellent body weight exercise that strengthens your legs and improves balance. Stand with your feet together, then step forward with one leg, lowering your hips until both knees are bent at 90-degree angles. Push back to the starting position and switch legs. Step-ups using a sturdy surface such as a bench or a set of stairs are also highly effective. Stand in front of the bench, step up with one foot, and bring the other foot up to meet it. Step back down and repeat with the opposite leg. This exercise targets your quads, hamstrings, and glutes while improving coordination.

To help you get started, here's a sample leg workout routine that can be completed in a short amount of time. Begin with three sets of 15 body weight squats. This exercise warms up your legs and engages multiple muscle groups. Next, perform three sets of 12 lunges, six on each leg. Lunges not only strengthen your legs but also improve your balance and coordination. Follow this with three sets of 10 step-ups, five on each leg. Step-ups are a great way to target your lower body and enhance functional mobility. Take a short rest between sets, about 30 seconds to one minute, to allow your muscles to recover.

As you progress and become more comfortable with these exercises, you can increase the difficulty of challenging your muscles. One way to do this is by adding pulses or holds at the bottom of a squat. For example, lower into a squat position and hold for a few seconds before standing back up. This increases the time your muscles are under tension, enhancing strength and endurance. Performing jump squats is another way to increase intensity. Start squatting and explode upwards, jumping as high as you can. Land softly and immediately lower back into the squat position. This plyometric movement adds cardio to your workout, boosting your heart rate and calorie burn. Incorporating single-leg variations, such as squats or step-ups, also intensifies the workout. These unilateral exercises require greater balance and coordination, further challenging your muscles.

By focusing on leg strength, you'll build a solid foundation that supports overall fitness and enhances daily activities. Strong legs are essential to improve athletic performance, reduce the risk of injury, or make everyday tasks easier. Incorporate these exercises into your routine, gradually increasing the difficulty of progressing. Your legs will become stronger, more resilient, and better equipped to support your active lifestyle.

Glutes and Thighs in 10 Minutes

When I started focusing on my lower body, I quickly realized the immense benefits of targeting the glutes and thighs. These muscle groups are not just about aesthetics; they play a crucial role in enhancing lower body strength, improving posture and balance, aiding in athletic performance, and contributing to overall body image. Strong glutes and thighs are the powerhouses that support many of our daily movements. These muscles are constantly at work, from sitting and standing to climbing stairs and running. Strengthening them can make everyday activities easier and more efficient.

A well-toned lower body improves posture and balance. The glutes, in particular, help stabilize the pelvis and maintain proper alignment of the spine. This stability reduces the risk of lower back pain and enables you to stand taller and move more gracefully. Improved posture not only enhances your physical appearance but also boosts your confidence. Additionally, strong glutes and thighs are essential for athletic performance. Whether you're sprinting, jumping, or lifting weights, these muscles provide the power and stability needed to perform at your best. They also help absorb the impact of high-intensity activities, reducing the risk of injury. Focusing on these muscle groups can significantly enhance your overall athletic abilities.

You don't need much time to target the glutes and thighs effectively. Here's a quick 10-minute routine that can help you build strength and tone these muscles. Start with one minute of glute bridges. Lie on your back with your knees bent and feet flat on the floor. Lift your hips towards the ceiling, squeezing your glutes at the top, and then lower back down. This exercise engages your glutes and hamstrings, helping to build strength and stability. Next, perform one minute of sumo squats. Stand with your feet wider than shoulder-width apart and your toes pointing outwards. Lower your body into a squat, keeping your knees aligned with your toes, and then push back up. This variation targets the inner thighs and glutes.

Move on to one minute of donkey kicks, 30 seconds per leg. Start on all fours with your hands directly under your shoulders and your knees under your hips. Lift one leg towards the ceiling, keeping your knee bent at 90 degrees, and lower it back down. This exercise isolates the glutes, providing an intense burn. Follow this with one minute of fire hydrants, 30 seconds per leg. In the same all-fours position, lift one leg to the side, keep your knee bent, and lower it back down. Fire hydrants target the gluteus medius, an essential muscle for hip stability. Finish the routine with two sets of one-minute wall sits. Find a wall and slide down until your thighs are parallel to the ground, holding this position. Wall sits engage the quadriceps, hamstrings, and glutes, helping to build endurance and strength.

Maintaining proper form and technique is crucial to maximize the benefits of these exercises and avoid injury. When performing squats, always keep your knees aligned with your toes to prevent unnecessary strain on your joints. During glute bridges, engage your core and avoid arching your back to protect your lower spine. For donkey kicks, focus on controlled movements and keep your back flat to ensure you're targeting the glutes effectively. Proper form ensures that you're working the intended muscles and getting the most out of your workout.

As you become more comfortable with these exercises, you can increase the difficulty of continuing to challenge your muscles. One way to do this is by adding resistance bands. Place a resistance band around your thighs for exercises like glute bridges and fire hydrants to increase the intensity. Performing single-leg glute bridges is another effective progression. Lift one leg off the ground and perform the glute bridge with the other leg, alternating sides. This unilateral movement challenges your stability and engages your core even more. You can also increase the duration or repetitions of each exercise. For example, extend the time of each exercise from one minute to 90 seconds or add more sets to your routine. These progressions ensure that your muscles grow more robust and more resilient over time.

By incorporating these exercises into your routine, you'll build stronger glutes and thighs, improving your overall fitness and enhancing your daily life. The benefits extend beyond aesthetics, contributing to better posture, balance, and athletic performance. With consistency and proper form, you'll see significant improvements in your lower body strength and endurance.

4.3 Low-Impact Lower Body Exercises for Seniors

When I started working with seniors, I noticed many hesitated to exercise due to joint pain and injury concerns. Low-impact exercises, however, offer a practical solution that can significantly improve quality of life. These exercises minimize joint strain, making them well-suited for seniors with arthritis or other joint problems. By focusing on gentle movements, seniors can enhance their mobility and flexibility without the risk of exacerbating existing conditions. This approach ensures that physical activity remains accessible and beneficial for everyone, regardless of age.

Low-impact exercises are also excellent for improving balance and stability. Our balance can deteriorate as we age, increasing the risk of falls and related injuries. By incorporating exercises that target balance, seniors can build the strength and coordination needed to navigate daily activities more safely. These exercises also help prevent injuries by strengthening the muscles around the joints, providing better support, and reducing the likelihood of falls. Enhanced balance and stability lead to greater confidence in movement, allowing seniors to maintain independence and enjoy a more active lifestyle.

Several low-impact exercises are particularly suitable for seniors. Seated leg lifts are a great starting point. Sit on a sturdy chair with a straight back and feet flat on the floor. Lift one leg straight before you, hold for a few seconds, then lower it back down. This exercise targets the quadriceps and helps improve leg strength. Standing calf raises are another effective exercise. Stand with your feet hip-width apart and hold onto the back of a chair for balance. Slowly rise onto your toes, hold briefly, then lower back down. Calf raises strengthen the calves and improve ankle stability. Chair squats are excellent for building leg strength without putting too much pressure on the knees. Stand in front of a chair with your feet shoulder-width apart. Lower your body as if you're going to sit down, then stand back up just before your bottom touches the chair. This movement engages the quads, hamstrings, and glutes. Side leg raises are also beneficial. Stand behind a chair and lift one leg to the side, keeping it straight. Lower it back down and repeat on the other side. This exercise targets the hip abductors and improves lateral stability.

To help you get started, here's a sample low-impact, lower-body workout routine. Begin with two sets of ten seated leg lifts, five per leg. This exercise will warm up your legs and gently engage your muscles. Next, perform two sets of fifteen standing calf raises. This movement strengthens your calves and improves balance. Follow this with two sets of ten-chair squats. Chair squats are a safe way to build leg strength and improve functional mobility. Finally, complete the routine with two sets of ten side leg raises, five per leg. This exercise targets the hip muscles and enhances lateral stability. Remember to take short breaks between sets to allow your muscles to recover.

Following safety tips and making necessary modifications are essential when performing these exercises. Always emphasize slow, controlled movements to ensure proper form and prevent injury. Using a chair or wall for balance support can provide additional stability and confidence, especially if you're new to exercise or have mobility issues. Avoid any exercises that cause pain or discomfort, and listen to your body. If an exercise feels too challenging, modify it to suit your abilities. For example, you can reduce the range of motion or perform fewer repetitions. Gradually increase the number of repetitions as your strength improves. This progressive approach ensures that you continue to make gains without overexerting yourself.

Low-impact exercises provide seniors with a safe and effective way to improve their lower body strength, mobility, and balance. By incorporating these gentle movements into your routine, you can enjoy the benefits of exercise while minimizing the risk of injury. With consistency and proper technique, you'll see significant improvements in your physical fitness and overall well-being.

4.4 Calf and Ankle Strengthening

I once struggled to keep my balance while navigating a rocky hiking trail. Then, I truly understood the importance of strong calves and ankles. These muscles play a crucial role in maintaining overall mobility and preventing injuries. Strengthening them supports your balance and stability, which is essential for everyday activities like walking, standing, and climbing stairs. When your calves and ankles are strong, you reduce the risk of ankle sprains, a common injury that can sideline you for weeks. Moreover, solid calves and ankles enhance athletic performance, providing the power needed for explosive movements such as running and jumping. Improved posture and gait are additional benefits, as these muscles help align your body correctly, making every step more efficient and reducing strain on other body parts.

Several practical exercises can help you strengthen your calves and ankles without equipment. Calf raises are a simple yet powerful exercise. Stand with your feet hip-width apart and slowly rise onto your toes, lifting your heels off the ground. Hold for a moment, then lower back down. This exercise targets the calf muscles, improving strength and endurance. Ankle circles are another great exercise. Sit down or stand on one leg, lift the other foot off the ground, and rotate your ankle in a circular motion. Perform this movement in both directions to ensure balanced development. Toe taps are also beneficial. While sitting or standing, lift your toes, keep your heels planted, and tap them back down. This exercise engages the muscles around your ankles, enhancing stability. Heel walks can further strengthen your calves and ankles. Walk on your heels for a set distance, keeping your toes off the ground. This movement targets the front part of your lower legs and improves balance.

Here's a structured routine focused on calf and ankle strengthening to get you started. Begin with three sets of 15 calf raises. This exercise will warm up your calf muscles and enhance their endurance. Next, perform three sets of 20 ankle circles, ten in each direction, to improve flexibility and strength around your ankles. Follow this with three sets of 15 toe taps, which target the muscles surrounding your ankles and enhance stability. Finish the routine with three sets of 30-second heel walks. This exercise strengthens your calves and improves your balance and coordination. Take short breaks between sets to allow your muscles to recover.

As your strength and confidence grow, you can increase the difficulty and effectiveness of these exercises. One way to do this is by performing single-leg calf raises. Instead of lifting both heels off the ground, lift one heel while balancing on the other foot. This unilateral movement challenges your balance and engages your core. Adding resistance bands to ankle exercises is another effective progression. For example, place a resistance band around your toes while performing ankle circles to increase the intensity. You can also increase the duration of heel walks. Instead of walking on your heels for 30 seconds, extend it to 60 seconds or more. These progressions ensure your muscles continue strengthening and adapting, providing better support and stability.

By focusing on calf and ankle strength, you build a solid foundation that supports overall mobility and prevents injuries. Whether you aim to enhance athletic performance, reduce the risk of ankle sprains, or improve your posture and gait, these exercises are key. Incorporate them into your routine, gradually increasing the difficulty to continue progressing. Your calves and ankles will become stronger, more resilient, and better equipped to support your active lifestyle.

In the next chapter, we will explore upper body strength, focusing on effective workouts that can be done quickly and efficiently. Building upper body strength is as important as lower body strength, which complements your work in this chapter. Let's continue our journey to a stronger, healthier you.

6

Chapter 5: Upper Body Strength

5.1 Arm Sculpting in 10 Minutes Arm strength is vital for daily tasks like lifting groceries and contributes to athletic performance. Declining muscle mass with age makes incorporating arm exercises into your fitness routine essential. A 10-minute arm workout can maintain strength, improve muscle tone, and enhance overall upper-body fitness. Begin with bicep curls using resistance bands or water bottles for one minute, followed by tricep dips on a chair for another minute. Proceed to one minute of arm circles, half a minute each for forward and backward circles. Continue with hammer curls to target the brachialis muscle for one minute, then move to overhead tricep extensions for another minute. Finish with two sets of alternating bicep and tricep exercises, each set lasting two minutes. Focus on proper form to avoid injury and maximize benefits—keep elbows close during curls and maintain core engagement throughout. Add weight or resistance, increase repetitions, or incorporate single-arm variations to progress. # 5.2 Quick Chest and Back Workouts Strong chest and back muscles are essential for posture, reducing back pain, and

33

enhancing stability. A 10-minute routine can significantly improve upper body strength. Start with one minute of push-ups, followed by chest flies using resistance bands or light weights for another minute. Then, do one minute of bent-over rows to strengthen the back, followed by the Superman exercise to target the lower back for another minute. Finish with chest presses for one minute and two sets of alternating chest and back exercises. Maintain a neutral spine during rows and keep your body straight during push-ups. For added intensity, perform knee push-ups if a beginner or add resistance bands to increase the challenge. # 5.3 Shoulder Workouts Without Weights Shoulder strength supports arm movements and contributes to upper body symmetry. A 10-minute no-equipment routine can enhance shoulder strength and endurance. Begin with shoulder taps from a plank position for one minute, followed by pike push-ups for another minute. Perform arm circles for one minute, transitioning from forward to backward circles. Continue with a plank to the downward dog for dynamic shoulder engagement, then finish with reverse plank shoulder stretches. Ensure proper alignment during push-up variations and keep shoulders down during arm circles. To increase difficulty, extend exercise duration, add resistance bands, or incorporate shoulder presses with household items. # 5.4 Push-Up Variations for All Levels Push-ups engage multiple upper body muscles, offering modifications for all fitness levels and improving endurance. Beginners can start with knee or wall push-ups, progressing to incline push-ups for a reduced load. Intermediate users can try wide-grip push-ups for the chest or diamond push-ups for the triceps. Advanced individuals can challenge themselves with decline push-ups, plyometric push-ups, or one-arm push-ups for increased intensity. Maintain a straight body line, engage the core, and keep elbows at a 45-degree angle during push-ups to target muscles effectively and prevent injury. Incorporating these exercises into your routine promotes upper body strength, endurance, and muscle tone, preparing you for high-intensity interval training (HIIT) designed for busy schedules.

7

Chapter 6: High-Intensity Interval Training (HIIT)

#**Quick Fit:** Efficient Workouts for Busy Lives After a draining day, the gym was the last thing on my mind. However, maintaining fitness was non-negotiable. That's when High-Intensity Interval Training (HIIT) came into play, revolutionizing how I approached exercise with its time-efficient routines. Introduction to HIIT High-Intensity Interval Training (HIIT) combines intense bursts of activity with brief rest periods, catering to various exercise preferences, from running to bodyweight exercises. Its adaptability ensures anyone can incorporate HIIT into their routine, benefiting from efficient calorie burn, improved cardiovascular health, and enhanced muscle tone within a 10-30 minute session. Research supports HIIT's efficacy, showing significant health improvements and a higher calorie burn rate post-exercise due to excess post-exercise oxygen consumption (EPOC).

Examples of Essential HIIT Exercises:

- Burpees and Jump Squats target multiple muscle groups, boosting cardiovascular endurance.

- Mountain Climbers and Sprints engage the core and elevate heart rate

- High knees improve cardio fitness and engage the core.

These exercises form the backbone of a HIIT routine, maximizing efficiency in minimal time. 15-Minute HIIT for Busy Professionals For those pressed for time, a 15-minute HIIT session can fit seamlessly into any schedule. A sample workout might include high knees, burpees, jump squats, and mountain climbers, interspersed with rest periods. This routine ensures a comprehensive workout targeting various muscle groups, emphasizing the importance of maintaining intensity and using time wisely with the help of timers or HIIT apps. Adapting HIIT for Various Environments HIIT's versatility allows for modifications in different settings, such as office spaces, homes, or outdoors, ensuring consistent workouts regardless of location. This adaptability makes HIIT an ideal solution for maintaining fitness amidst a busy lifestyle. Low-Impact HIIT for Beginners Low-impact HIIT offers a gentler approach suitable for beginners or those with joint concerns. Exercises like marching in place, seated leg lifts, and step touches provide a vigorous workout without the high-impact stress, making fitness accessible and sustainable. Advanced HIIT Challenges For the seasoned fitness enthusiast, advanced HIIT routines introduce more complex exercises like plyometric push-ups and pistol squats, pushing physical and mental boundaries. Equipment like kettlebells or battle ropes can further intensify these workouts, promoting muscle growth and endurance.

In conclusion, HIIT's flexibility and time efficiency make it a valuable exercise mode for individuals at any fitness level. Whether squeezing a session into a hectic day or pushing your limits with advanced routines, HIIT offers a practical path to achieving and maintaining peak physical health. Next, we'll explore the importance of flexibility and mobility exercises to complement your HIIT regimen, keeping your fitness journey balanced and injury-free.

8

Chapter 7: Flexibility and Mobility

On Quick Workouts: A Guide for Busy Lives Quick workouts are not merely a convenience; they're a transformative approach to fitness that meshes with the complexities of modern life. These concise yet potent workouts offer a means to enhance health without overtaking one's schedule. From a brisk ten-minute session to a more extended thirty-minute dive, these exercises afford flexibility, energy, and strength necessary for daily endeavors. This exploration begins with the foundational elements of quick workouts, emphasizing the necessity of warm-ups and cooldowns to prime the body for activity and facilitate recovery. Core strength, lower body power, and upper body fortification are broken down to provide specific and time-efficient exercises. The merits of High-Intensity Interval Training (HIIT) are unveiled, showcasing its capacity to optimize calorie expenditure and bolster cardiovascular health within compressed time frames. Flexibility and mobility are spotlighted as pivotal to a holistic fitness regimen, ensuring fluid, pain-free movement. Cardio and strength training synthesis emerges as a cornerstone strategy, adaptable to varying fitness levels and settings. The significance of monitoring progress and maintaining motivation is addressed, introducing tools like progress mazes and fitness journals for engagement and accountability. Focusing on safety and injury prevention, the narrative highlights the significance of maintaining proper form and technique. With actionable meal timing and composition advice, nutrition's role in supporting workout efficacy and recovery is detailed. Quick workouts exemplify efficiency and adaptability, proving that consistency trumps duration. Embracing these principles, even the busiest individuals can weave exercise into their daily lives, fostering health, energy, and resilience. Aligned with these physical endeavors, nutrition amplifies results, underscoring the symbiotic relationship between diet and exercise. As you embark on your fitness journey, remember the power and potential of quick workouts. They offer a sustainable, flexible path to fitness, one that accommodates the demands of modern life while promoting health and well-being. Keep exploring, stay motivated, and embrace the journey towards a stronger, healthier self.

I hope you found this book to be helpful. I would appreciate it if you left a favorable review for the book on Amazon.

9

Conclusion

In conclusion, *Quick Fit* proves that achieving your fitness goals doesn't require hours at the gym. This guide empowers you to integrate efficient, high-impact exercises into your daily routine, no matter how busy your schedule.

With its focus on short yet effective workouts, practical advice, and motivating success stories, *Quick Workouts* offers a clear path to better health and fitness. You'll learn how to maximize your time, stay motivated, and make fitness a natural part of your life.

Take control of your well-being and experience the benefits of a fitter, healthier you. Embrace the simplicity and effectiveness of quick workouts today, and let this book be your companion on the journey to a more active and fulfilling lifestyle. Start your transformation now and see how a few minutes a day can make a difference!

References

- Evidence-Based Effects of High-Intensity Interval Training ... https://www.ncbi.nlm.nih.gov/pmc/articles/PMC8294064/
- *Effects of one long vs. two short resistance training ...* https://www.ncbi.nlm.nih.gov/pmc/articles/PMC9557220/
- *How Even Super-Short Workouts Can Improve Your Health* https://time.com/6242876/short-workouts-health-benefits/
- *How SMART Fitness Goals Can Help You Get Healthier* https://health.clevelandclinic.org/smart-fitness-goals
- *Warm Up, Cool Down* https://www.heart.org/en/healthy-living/fitness/fitness-basics/warm-up-cool-down
- *A 9-Minute Warm-Up Routine Before Your Workout* https://www.nytimes.com/2024/07/11/well/move/workout-warm-up-exercise.html
- *Cool down Exercises: 16 Ways to Cool Down with Instructions*

https://www.healthline.com/health/exercise-fitness/cool down-exercises

- *Static and Dynamic Stretching: Tips for Athletes* https://www.hss.edu/article_static_dynamic_stretching.asp
- *This 5-Minute Core Workout Will Help You Build Your ...* https://www.mindbodygreen.com/articles/this-5-minute-core-workout-will-help-you-build-your-strength-asap
- *15 Plank Variations Your Core Will Thank You for Later* https://www.healthline.com/health/14-plank-variations-your-core-will-thank-you-for-later
- *The 9 Best Ab Exercises You Can Do Without ...* https://us.myprotein.com/thezone/training/best-ab-exercises-you-can-do-without-equipment/
- *Beginner Core Workout: 10 Pilates Ab Exercises for ...* https://www.today.com/health/diet-fitness/beginner-core-workout-rcna29378
- *The Importance of Leg Strength to Overall Health* https://coloradopaincare.com/the-importance-of-leg-strength-to-overall-health/
- *31 Leg Exercises at Home That Require No Equipment* https://www.self.com/gallery/killer-legs-no-gear-required-slideshow
- *13 Glute Exercises: Benefits of Working Your Glutes - 2024* https://www.masterclass.com/articles/glute-workouts
- *12 Leg Strengthening Exercises for Seniors to Reduce Falls* https://holidayretirement.com/easy-leg-exercises-for-seniors-to-improve-mobility/
- *Everyday arm exercises: Functional benefits - Harvard Health* https://www.health.harvard.edu/exercise-and-fitness/everyday-arm-exercises-functional-benefits#:~:text=Strong%20arms%20aren't%20just,strength%2C%20espe-

cially%20as%20we%age.

- *A 10-Minute Arms Workout for Stronger Biceps, Triceps, ...* https://www.self.com/gallery/10-minute-arms-workout-watching-tv
- *How to Do Triceps Dips: Techniques, Benefits, Variations* https://www.verywellfit.com/the-chair-dip-triceps-exercise-3120734
- *16 Push-Up Variations to Build Strength for Every Fitness ...* https://www.shape.com/fitness/workouts/arm-workouts/push-up-variations
- *Evidence-Based Effects of High-Intensity Interval Training ...* https://www.ncbi.nlm.nih.gov/pmc/articles/PMC8294064/
- *HIIT Workouts for Beginners | Starter HIIT Exercises* https://www.puregym.com/blog/hiit-workouts-for-beginners/
- *A 15-Minute HIIT Workout You Can Do With Just Your ...* https://www.self.com/gallery/15-minute-hiit-workout
- *The Best Low-Impact HIIT Exercises for Joint-Friendly Fitness* https://www.hitonefitness.com/the-best-low-impact-hiit-exercises-for-joint-friendly-fitness/
- *The importance of stretching* https://www.health.harvard.edu/staying-healthy/the-importance-of-stretching
- *Yoga for Flexibility: 8 Poses for Your Back, Core, Hips ...* https://www.healthline.com/health/exercise-fitness/yoga-for-flexibility
- *5 Joint Mobility Exercises to Improve Flexibility and Function* https://www.healthline.com/health/fitness-exercise/joint-mobility-exercises
- *Best Pilates Exercises To Improve Your Flexibility* https://evergreenclinic.ca/best-pilates-exercises-to-improve-your-fle

xibility/

- *Combining Strength Training and Cardio May Help Longevity* https://www.health.com/combining-strength-training-cardio-longevity-6748178
- *Effective 20-Minute, Full-Body Workout You Can Do at Home* https://www.verywellfit.com/20-minute-full-body-workout-exercises-and-tips-6560761
- *Why Having Proper Form & Exercise Techniques is Important* https://jackcityfitness.com/why-having-proper-fitness-form-technique-is-important/
- *Making Workouts Work For You: How To Modify Exercises* https://www.anytimefitness.com/ccc/how-to/how-to-modify-exercises/
- *Navigating the Maze: Your Ultimate Guide to Healthy Weight ...* https://atrustednurse.com/2024/03/08/navigating-the-maze-your-ultimate-guide-to-healthy-weight-management/
- *The Benefits of Keeping a Fitness Journal* https://columbiaassociation.org/gyms-fitness/the-benefits-of-keeping-a-fitness-journal/
- *How SMART Fitness Goals Can Help You Get Healthier* https://health.clevelandclinic.org/smart-fitness-goals
- *Need Some Workout Motivation? Check Out These Stories* https://www.brickbodies.com/need-workout-motivation-check-inspiring-stories/
- *Why Having Proper Form & Exercise Techniques is Important* https://jackcityfitness.com/why-having-proper-fitness-form-technique-is-important/
- *Workout Injuries: Prevention and Treatment* https://www.webmd.com/fitness-exercise/workout-injuries-prevention-and-treatment

- *Making Workouts Work For You: How To Modify Exercises* https://www.anytimefitness.com/ccc/how-to/how-to-modify-exercises/
- *How to Listen to Your Body While Exercising, Eating, and …* https://www.fitnessblender.com/articles/how-to-listen-to-your-body-while-exercising-eating-and-in-times-of-stress-improve-your-relationship
- *Pre-Workout Nutrition: What to Eat Before a Workout* https://www.healthline.com/nutrition/eat-before-workout
- *Post-Workout Nutrition: What to Eat After a Workout* https://www.healthline.com/nutrition/eat-after-workout
- *Sports and Hydration for Athletes: Q&A with a Dietitian* https://www.hopkinsmedicine.org/health/wellness-and-prevention/nutrition-and-fitness/sports-and-hydration-for-athletes
- *The Ultimate Meal Plan Guide for the Busy Millennial* https://prettysimpledays.com/2020/02/15/the-ultimate-meal-plan-guide-for-the-busy-millennial/
- *The Complete 4-Week Beginner's Workout Program* https://www.muscleandfitness.com/workout-plan/workouts/workout-routines/complete-mf-beginners-training-guide-plan/
- *Strength Progressions for Beginner and Intermediate Lifters* https://www.elitefts.com/education/strength-progressions-for-beginner-and-intermediate-lifters/
- *Advanced HIIT Workout - Total Body High-Intensity Interval …* https://www.fitnessblender.com/videos/advanced-hiit-workout-total-body-high-intensity-interval-training
- *7 Low Impact Exercises for Older Adults to Stay Active* https://www.humangood.org/resources/senior-living

REFERENCES

-blog/low-impact-exercises-for-older-adults